# Low Carb Diet

*The Best Guide To Low Carb - Lose Fat And Get A Fast Metabolism In 7 Days With This Weight Loss Blood Sugar Solution Diet!*

**Chris Smith**

Copyright © 2013 Chris Smith

## STOP!!! Before you read any further....Would you like to know the Secrets of Body Transformation?

If your answer is yes, then you are not alone. Thousands of people are looking for the secret to rapidly burn body fat, keep the weight off, become healthier, and truly transform their body and life for good.

If you have been searching for these answers without much luck, you are in the right place!

Not only will you gain incredible insight in this book, but because I want to make sure to give you as much value as possible, right now for a limited time you can get full **100% FREE access to a VIP bonus EBook** entitled **THE 7 KEYS TO BODY TRANSFORMATION!**

## Just Go Here For Free Instant Access:

## www.liveFitVIP.com

# Legal Notice

# Disclaimer Notice

## Table Of Contents

# Introduction

I want to thank you and congratulate you for purchasing the book, *"Low Carb Diet: The Best Guide To Low Carb - Lose Fat And Get A Fast Metabolism In 7 Days With This Weight Loss Blood Sugar Solution Diet!"*.

This book contains proven steps and strategies on how to get the body of your dreams!

Don't let another week pass you by living life out of shape! The extra weight around your waistline or hips is more than just a problem of how you look in the mirror. Especially if it is not burned off in the near future, it can cause a host of other problems relating to your health and longevity. You owe it to yourself and the ones close to you to get in the best shape of your life.

Imagine how nice it would feel to look in the mirror and be happy with what you see on the outside and be comforted knowing that you are much healthier on the inside.

If you are serious about finally losing weight and keeping it off, then you have come to the right place. "Low Carb Diet: Low Carb Diet Solution - In as Little as 7 Days You Can Lose Weight Fast Using This Low Carb Diet Plan!" is the solution you have been looking for that allows you to literally create the body of your dreams, and what's even better is you will start seeing results within the first 7 days. Anyone who truly wants to lose weight can use these principles and be on their way in a matter of days! Don't waste another week, begin living life to the fullest today!

This book does not offer a drastic solution. But it will show you how to customize your low carb meals for seven days so you can start experiencing your desired weight loss results.

Thanks again for purchasing this book, I hope you enjoy it!

# Chapter 1 – What Is A Low Carb Diet?

I am so excited for you! If you are reading this far, it means that you truly are looking for change in your life! You are tired of not living to your full potential, and ready to start living the way you were intended to. That's great, and what better way to start than by creating the best body of your life!

Keep that enthusiasm high because that is exactly what will carry you through to reaching your goals. The truth is the most important factor in your goals being obtained is you. You are the one that must "decide". You must simply make a choice that no matter what, you will reach your goal. If you simply do this, than I am confident you will succeed.

So let's get started! But Before we jump straight into what you should eat and the details of the diet, we need to make sure you are caught up to speed on the basics of a low carb diet.

If you've been dieting or have at least tried to do something about your weight, then you might have heard or read about low carb diets. Some of the popular fad-diets that can be classified as low carb diets include Sugar Busters Diet, the well-known South Beach Diet, the ever popular Zone Diet, Atkins, and pretty much every other diet you may have heard of

As you should know by now, the term "low carb diet" has actually been applied to many different diets. It's a really broad classification of different diets that limit carbohydrate intake. Some people call them low glycemic diets while others refer to them as reduced carbohydrate diets.

The common denominator for these diets that belong to the "low carb" class is that they require, just as the name suggests, a diet that excludes foods that are heavy in carbohydrates. These are foods that are referred to as glycemic. There are lists of foods and their glycemic index to guide people going on any low carb diet.

So How Low Carb is Low Carb, Really?

You may consult your doctor about how low carb your diet should be; this is the smartest thing you should do before engaging in any diet. The dietary guidelines in the United States state that around 50 to 65 percent of a person's calorie intake for any given day should come from carbs.

Generally speaking, you should simply have less than 50% to 65% calories coming from carbohydrate sources of any variant in your daily diet. There are low carb diets that recommend only 20% or less of your daily caloric intake. If you want to live off a low carb diet for weight loss, keeping your carbohydrate intake to less than 20% of your daily caloric requirement is advised. Of course, you should make sure that you substitute this with another calorie source, mostly vegetables. With this kind of drastic drop in carbohydrate consumption, not all people are able to handle the dietary changes.

Your body will react. You can feel uneasy because of cravings for the carbs that you are used to having. That is why you will have to slowly adjust your carb intake up to the point when your body can take the loss of carbs. You may think that's a bit of a hit and miss approach, but the fact remains that everyone has a different tolerance for carb loss.

# Chapter 2 – Different Approaches To Achieve Ideal Results

Notice that different low carb diets will use different approaches to achieve the desired effects. One approach is to simply just reduce a person's carb intake immediately. The idea behind this approach is pretty basic: the fewer carbs you take in the fewer calories you gain, period.

If you count calories and check out the numbers, then this approach may sound very plausible. These kinds of diets usually advise against adding sugars or using refined carb sources.

The methodology is simple. All you have to do is to get rid of the side orders, extra helpings, and meal add-ons in your diet that tend to bloat your calorie intake. Another way to apply this approach is to simply get rid of the white foods you usually eat like white flour, white refined sugar, rice and any other white grains, and potatoes (white or yellow ones included).

The next approach is to determine just how much carbs each dieter needs to take off his meals in order to lose weight. This method is less drastic and a lot safer for people. It follows the idea that each person has a different carb tolerance. Older people have a harder time digesting carbs. The objective in this approach is to define the optimal carb level for each individual. This is basically one of the ideas behind the South Beach Diet and similar diets.

The last approach is to teach your body to use the calories from stores in your body fat. Your body is naturally attuned to using fat in order to gain energy. It will take time for your body to stop making use of glucose and concentrate on the use of stored fat in the body. This process is called ketosis.

Diets that make use of this bodily process are called ketonic diets. Note that some ketonic diets are applied by some medical experts to treat chronic diseases such as epilepsy. However, when this approach is applied to weight loss, it is referred to by such experts as James Volek and Stephen Phinneyas nutritional ketosis. One of the phases of the Atkins diet is actually ketogenic in nature. This approach is not suited for everyone, but there are people who have become quite successful at losing weight using ketonic diets.

During the initial stages of ketosis the brain will refrain from burning ketones. Doing so, the body will stop making use of stored glycogen but will instead concentrate on making use of stored body fat. In this mode, your body will make use of stored carbs only when it is absolutely necessary. This also helps prevent your body from eating up the stored proteins found in your muscles.

# Chapter 3 – The Case Of The Atkins Diet: To Be Strict Or Not

In this Chapter, we'll look into one of the low carb diets that have become popular in recent years, the Atkins Diet. We'll look into its pros and cons and we'll allow you to decide if it is the right one for you.

The Atkins Diet has four stages or phases: Induction, Ongoing Weight Loss, Pre-Maintenance, and Maintenance. There is no set pattern on which phase one should start with. However, it is highly encouraged that people begin with the Induction Phase since it will prepare the body for the drop in carbohydrates. This is also the phase where ketosis occurs since your body will be induced or forced into burning fat stores rather than glycogen stores.

Looking Into the Induction Phase

This Phase will help you figure out your carb tolerance level. Once you know how many carbs you can basically live with, the diet will then adjust to how your body behaves. You will have to determine how much carbs you can bear losing. Once that level is determined, dieters will then monitor carb intake and maintain the level where they are able to successfully lose weight. The Induction lasts for a period of two weeks but staying on it longer is also encouraged.

Foods Allowed

Dieters going through the Atkins diet should avoid refined sources of carbs. You can eat any carb source that is nutrient dense. Just like any low carb diet out there, the emphasis in food choice has to do with smartly choosing your sources of carbohydrates.

Dieters are supposed to get most of their carbs from vegetables. Dieters are allowed 12 to 15 grams of vegetables each day. They are also allowed to consume protein as well as fats. Most types of cheeses are allowed, but not fresh cheeses such as farmer's cheese or cottage cheese. Dieters are allowed only three to four ounces of cheese each day.

Protein sources such as eggs, meat, and seafood are okay. You are also allowed to eat plenty of omega 3 fatty acid sources (e.g. cold water fish etc.). Olive oil, grape seed oil, peanut oil, and canola oil are also allowed. Surprisingly, regular full fat mayonnaise is allowed as well as butter.

When it comes to beverages, water is number one (this is basically the case for any low carb diet). Any beverage that has sugar in it is not allowed. However, diet sodas that are sweetened using Splenda (sucralose) are allowed. Splenda and Sweet n Low (saccharine) are your basic sweeteners while on this diet. Low carb snacks are allowed but you should check the label for sugar content.

The Pros and Cons of the Induction Phase

The induction phase of the Atkins Diet has received a lot of negative criticism even from proponents of low carb dieting. They cite the fact that it is too restrictive. If you look at the earlier books on the Atkins Diet, they stress this phase as an extremely important part of the Diet. Nowadays, however, Atkins Diet authors tend to veer away from such assertions.

The good side of this phase is that it jump starts you into the very heart of low carb dieting. You'll be giving up a lot of carbs in the onset. If you are used to eating a lot of carbs, then this phase will allow you to make a 180 degree turn towards the other direction. It sort of drastically changes your eating habits right smack into what healthy eating should be.

On the bad side, this diet presents a radical dietary change that might not be tolerable for some people. However, experts say that you can actually start on a carb level that is higher than what the Induction Phase recommends. You can simply work on a gradual decrease of carbohydrates as you progress in the diet.

More Pros and Cons of Low Carb Diets

Aside from possibly getting a carb crashas mentioned above, there are some other negatives about the Atkins Diet that you should know about. As it has come under scrutiny, you might have heard about a number of both positive and negative things about it, including myths and misconceptions.

One of the popular comments about the Atkins Diet is that counting carbs is a meticulous process which requires a lot of planning. Once you have gotten the hang of low carb meal planning, however, you will not have to do a lot of counting anymore.

Boredom is another common negative among all low carb diets. With very few food choices, some people eventually get bored with the diet. The answer to this is a lot of creativity in meal options and low carb recipes.

Moving on to the positive side of this diet, people who love their steak and butter will be happy to note that these foods that are often forbidden in other diets are back on the menu. While this diet is restrictive when it comes to carbs and sugars, it is actually quite lenient on the other tasty treats that you normally crave for. That being said, it should be noted that dieters are still supposed to consume a variety of fats, which include healthy fats such as the ones from olive oil etc.

The Atkins Diet as well as other low carb diets is pretty easy to learn. Once you learn how to count carbs and identify the foods you can eat, you don't have to think much about everything else. Another good thing about low carb diets in general is that you are encouraged to find your own carbohydrate sensitivity. You get to determine just how much carbs you need to remove from your diet and how much you can tolerate.

# Chapter 4 – What Does A Low Carb Diet Look Like?

So, what does a low carb diet meal look like? The following are breakfast options, lunch options, dinner options, and snack options that you will find in many low carb diet plans. If you want to try living a slightly low carb diet than the one you're in right now, I suggest that you plan your meals for 7 days and choose from the following options.

## Breakfast Options

The following are breakfast options that you can mix and match. You will still be able to have bread, eggs, and cereals for breakfast. The big difference is that they won't be that heavy in their carb content.

*Breads:* bread, muffins, or biscuits made from low carb ingredients such as almond meal or flax meal. If you miss pancakes, you can find low carb pancake mixes too.

*Low Carb Cereals:* choose high fiber cereals like Fiber One. Check the label and make sure that cereals you choose are truly low carb.

*Eggs:* The easiest way to cook eggs is to boil them. Note that one hardboiled egg contains 0.5 grams of net carbs. But that is not always a tasty treat. To add flavor to eggs, turn them into an omelet with some left over veggies tossed into the mix.

*Low Carb Fruit Breakfast:* Fruits are a great low carb breakfast option. Examples of which include blackberries, cranberries, and lemons. The following fruits have medium sugar content: peaches, grapefruit, strawberries, apricots, papaya, guavas, cantaloupes, apples, casaba melons, honeydew melons, water melons, blueberries, and nectarines.

Now there are fruits that have higher sugar content, so be careful with these: pineapple, pears, plums, kiwifruit, and oranges. The following fruits should rarely be eaten. If you do, you should reduce your carb intake from other sources. The fruits with high sugar content are as follows: bananas, tangerines, mangoes, cherries, figs, and grapes.

*Spoonable Breakfasts:* Let's face it. There are mornings when you'll be in a hurry and won't have time to prepare a low carb meal. You can go pick some of the fruit mentioned above and you can add some of the following: ricotta cheese, yogurt, and cottage cheese. That's a pretty tasty quick breakfast you can spoon to your heart's content.

## Lunch Ideas

Lunch is one of the important meals of the day. It's your mid-way break in your eight hour work day or school day. Lunches are often done in a hurry. Those who do not have time to prepare their lunch would be constrained to go for fast food which normally consists of a burger, a big-sized soda, and some fries on the side. This lunch is eaten just as fast as it is ordered. It does not take a dietitian to say that this is not healthy at all.

You basically have to try to deviate from the usual lunch ideas and stick to healthier food choices that are low in carbs. You'll get the energy that you need to complete your day without loading up on the fats that make you gain weight. The options below will give you a lot to choose from when planning your week's lunches. They are relatively easy to prepare and they taste just as good as any good old lunch you ever had.

Salad not Sandwich

Many people grew up with the idea of having sandwiches for lunch. A couple of slices of white bread with veggies and meat in between would have been the perfect lunch if you're not overweight. If you're trying to lose weight, you better skip the white bread and stick to the stuff sandwiched in the middle.

Go with veggies, cheese, and meat. When you think about it, this suggestion sounds more like a salad. Salads are the best way to go when you're making lunch on the go even if you're on a low carb diet.

*Salad Options:* The most common salad option is the good old chef's salad: one serving of iceberg lettuce (the size of a tennis ball) chopped, one hardboiled egg, chopped cold cuts, and a sprinkle of cheese. That already looks great and it's a great weight loss option too. However, it won't be too appetizing if you have that for lunch every day for seven days.

The good news is that there are a lot of salad options for lunch when you're on a low carb diet. When choosing salad greens, it is better to go for the darker greens. They are definitely more nutritious. At least you know which kind of bagged greens you're supposed to get from the grocery store.

A bunch of leaves with spices and a few other vegetables don't make a mean salad. What really makes a salad a true blue salad is the dressing. However, not every dressing will work wonders for your low carb diet. The following salad dressings will work best for your low carb diet plan:

*Caesar Salad Dressing:* 0.5 gram net carbs

*Oil and Vinegar:* 1 gram net carbs

*Ranch:* 1.4 grams net carbs

*Blue Cheese:* 2.3 grams net carbs

*Lime Juice:* 2.8 grams net carbs

*Lemon Juice:* 2.8 grams net carbs

Italian Dressing: 3 grams net carbs

NOTE: All servings on this list are 2 tablespoons. Don't add sugar to dressing.

With the many salad greens as well as dressing options available you can make the following salads: Thai chicken salad, Greek salad, tuna salad, chopped salad with chicken, blanched greens with salmon, and low carb taco salad among many others.

*Slightly Heavier Lunch Options:* There are folks who want a slightly heavier lunch, which is understandable if you're going on a low carb diet for the very first time. There are lunch options that are great for dieters who want to avoid a lot of carbs.

The following are some of your best lunch options for heavier low carb meals:

Baked salmon (200 grams), snow peas, spring greens, and a drizzle of lemon juice.

Diced seasonal veggies (1 cup), miso soup (225 ml).

Grilled chicken (180 grams) with a light drizzle of fresh squeezed lemon juice, whole grain rice (1 cup).

One serving of miso soup (300 ml), grilled tofu and bokchoy (100 grams).

Baked chicken (180 grams without skin) with vinaigrette flavoring (15 ml).

Canned tuna (95 grams), diced onions, lettuce (1 cup), and lemon zest.

Sourdough (1 piece), scrambled eggs (2 pieces), half a cup diced tomatoes.

Cooked quinoa (1 cup), steamed broccoli (one cup), walnuts (10 grams).

Pan fried steak (5 ounces), mushroom (1 cup) plus herbs, steamed green beans (1 cup).

Burgers (minus the buns); you can go to your favorite burger place, order bun-less burgers or just remove the burgers yourself. Don't get any extra orders on the side like French fries or onion rings and you shouldn't get any sweetened drink – just water will do.

## Dinner Options

Dinners can be tempting especially if you have your carb reduced dishes served alongside what the rest of the family is eating. Sometimes, losing weight is a lonely enterprise. You need the help and support of the entire family especially come dinner time when all of you are gathered around the dinner table. If you're lucky enough to get the family on the same ground, you can all have the same low carb meal during dinner.

The following are tasty dinner options that are definitely low carb. They are delectable enough so that the rest of the family can enjoy the same dishes with you. You can create your meal plans for an entire week and pick from any of the dishes mentioned here.

Baked Meatballs

You only need half a pound each of ground pork, ground round, and ground lamb. You'll also need one egg, chopped spinach (5 ounces), 1 teaspoon garlic (minced), 1 teaspoon salt, 1 teaspoon dried basil, half a teaspoon of crushed pepper, and half a cup of bread crumbs.

You just have to mix everything up, except for the bread crumbs of course. Place the mixture in the fridge and leave it there for 24 hours. Take it out the next evening, preheat your oven to 400 degrees Fahrenheit. Turn the mixture into 1.5 ounce balls, roll them over the bread crumbs, place them on a sheet, and bake them for 20 minutes. You can place the balls in individual muffin cups if you like.

One serving will have about four meatballs. It only yields 10 grams of carbs! This meal also provides you with 432 calories. Now, even your kids won't complain about this low carb menu item.


Spaghetti Squash

There's always room for spaghetti in low carb menus. You'll be cooking spaghetti the same old way except that instead of using the usual pasta you're going to use spaghetti squash, which has lower carb content. Regular pasta will give you 42 grams of carbs per serving while spaghetti squash will only yield 10 grams of carbs per serving. You will also have a full tummy with just 42 calories in your spaghetti squash low carb dinner.

## Cauliflower Chowder

This is not a pure cauliflower recipe, so you don't have to worry about stuffing yourself with a single veggie. You'll need five slices of bacon (chopped), onion powder (1 teaspoon), 1 stalk of celery (chopped), water (2 tablespoons), flour (2 tablespoons), salt and pepper, shredded cauliflower (4 cups), shredded cheddar cheese (12 ounces), 2 chopped green onions, and 2 cups of chicken broth.

Mix together one quarter chicken broth plus flour and set it aside. Sauté bacon, and place on paper towels when crispy to remove excess fat. Sauté onions, garlic, and celery; season with salt and pepper.

After that, you can add the cauliflower, chicken broth, water, and milk, and bring it to a boil. Add in the flour and chicken broth mixture and simmer for 3 minutes or until the chowder has thickened. You may then add the bacon and cheddar cheese. You can top the chowder with either drops of hot sauce or chopped green onions.

This recipe makes a total of eight servings. It only provides seven grams of carbs and it makes a very satisfying dinner.

Other Dinner Ideas: There are a lot of low carb dinner ideas to come and you definitely won't miss the carbs once you're full these really tasty and satisfying foods. Here are some more dinner ideas for low carb diets:

- Baked salmon (200 grams)
- Canned tuna (95 grams)
- Grilled chicken (180 grams)
- Grilled tofu (100 grams)
- Grilled trout (200 grams)
- Mixed beans salad

## Veggie Food Options

When you're going for a 7 day low carb menu plan, you should replace the bulk of the carbs you usually eat with veggies. It is recommended that you consume around 12 to 15 grams of net carbs coming from vegetables. A serving would be about the size of a tennis ball. Here are some quick bits of info that you can use when preparing veggies for your meals:

- Alfalfa sprouts: serving size 16 grams; 0.2 g net carbs
- Asparagus: serving size 6 spears; 2.4 g net carbs
- Artichoke hearts: serving size 1 can; 1 g net carbs
- Broccoli: serving size 80 grams; 1.7 g net carbs
- Celery: serving size 1 stalk; 0.4 g net carbs
- Chives: serving size 1 tablespoon; 0.1 g net carbs
- Cauliflower: serving size 60 grams; 1.4 net carbs
- Bok Choy: serving size 70 grams; 0.4 g net carbs
- Iceberg lettuce: serving size 70 grams; 0.2 g net carbs
- Romaine lettuce: serving size 45 grams; 0.4 g net carbs
- Mushrooms: serving size 35 grams; 1.2 g net carbs
- Kale: serving size 65 grams; 2.4 g net carbs
- Leeks: serving size 50 grams; 3.4 g net carbs
- Green string beans: serving size 100 grams; 4.1 g net carbs
- Green olives: serving size 5 pieces; 0.1 g net carbs
- Black olives: serving size 5 pieces; 0.7 g net carbs
- Sauerkraut: serving size 70 grams; 1.2 g net carbs
- Onion: serving size 20 grams; 4.3 g net carbs
- Spaghetti squash: serving size 40 grams when boiled; 2.0 g net carbs
- Okra: serving size 80 grams; 2.4 g net carbs
- Spinach: serving size 90 grams; 2.2 g net carbs
- Snow peas: serving size 60 grams; 3.4 g net carbs
- Tomatoes: serving size 60 grams; 4.3 g net carbs

Snack Options

In case you find yourself hungry at any point in your low carb dieting, you may want to gobble up some snacks to curb the craving without putting on more carbs. You may include any of the following in your meal plans:

- One apple + 10 cashews
- 1 banana + 10 cashews

- One banana + 5 Brazil nuts
- Liver cleanse juice (ginger root, beetroot, ½ regular size carrot, and celery)
- 10 cashews
- 30grams of hummus + 1 piece of unrefined whole wheat pita bread
- 30grams of mixed dried fruit (watch the sugar content)
- 1 whole wheat pita with ¼ avocado
- One regular sized banana
- 1 orange + 5 Brazil nuts (just have to love Brazil)
- 30grams hummus + carrot sticks
- 1 chopped carrot + 4 olives
- Banana Strawberry Shake (cheat treat – use only once a week!)

# Chapter 5 – How To Make Your 7 Day Low Carb Meal Plan

This is the point where you will make sense of it all. In the previous chapter you have been given a list of food items, meals, and recipes that you can make in order to get you started on a low carb diet.

The next step is to make a meal plan for days one to seven. Choose a breakfast option for each of the seven days. Choose a lunch option for each day. And choose a lunch option for each day.

The 6 Hour Secret

Now, the idea is to not go hungry within a six hour period. You're used to eating lots of carbs during the day and a good strategy to help you overcome any hunger pangs and cravings is to have low carb snacks ready for consumption within any six hour period.

When it comes to snacks, you can just wing it or make a schedule just like what you did for breakfast, lunch, and dinner. Have a good low carb drink ready in a drink bottle so you don't get tempted to grab a can of soda or any sugary drink. If you must sweeten your drink, make sure that you use Splenda (sucralose) or Sweet n Low (saccharine).

Sample Single Day Meal Plan

> Breakfast: Sourdough toast (1 slice only) + 50 grams of ricotta; drizzle with 2 tablespoons honey

> Snack: Carrot sticks and hummus

> Lunch: Canned tuna (95 grams) + diced lemons and lettuce

> Snack: 30 grams mixed dried fruit + cashews (10 pieces)

> Dinner: Grilled chicken (180 grams) with steamed broccoli.

> Drinks during the day: tea (sweetened with Splenda if desired), water (eight glasses)

# Conclusion

Thank you again for purchasing this book on the best way to implement a Low Carb Diet in your eating program!

I hope this book was able to help you to gain insights about the principles of a low carb diet and the strategies that you can use to achieve the body that you have been dreaming of.

The next step is to get started!

The tips in this book won't give you drastic results. What you have been given are flexible and doable strategies to get you started on a low carb diet. Putting these strategies to practice is up to you. How dedicated you are with your diet strategies will determine your success. The low carb diet works, but only if you stick to what it requires.

Once you are comfortable with the lenient and easy to follow low carb strategy described in this book, you can move on to more restrictive diets if you wish to achieve faster results. The important thing is to condition your body to a low carb diet or at least a semi-restricted carb diet. Once you have taken that first step, you can move on to further weight loss using more stringent low carb diet solutions.

Finally, if you enjoyed this book, please take the time to share your thoughts and post a review on Amazon. It'd be greatly appreciated!

Thank you and good luck!

# Preview Of:

# Fat Loss Secrets

## *No Diets, No Supplements, Just Fat Loss Truth!*

# Introduction

I want to thank you and congratulate you for purchasing the book, *"Fat Loss Secrets - No Diets, No Supplements, Just Fat Loss Truth!"*

This book contains proven steps and strategies on how to lose fat and get the body you have always dreamed of!

Over the years, countless fad diets have come and gone. Along with the fad diets came the supplements. At first, some of the supplements seemed like they could be of benefit to you and healthy for you to consume, but as time has gone on so has the supplement industry. Supplements are now chemically engineered magic potion pills. Some of them do help you lose body fat, but at what expense to your health?

It doesn't have to be this complicated! If you are tired of riding the diet roller coaster and jumping on and off the hope train of the supplement industry, then you have come to the right place. This is where, armored with the truth, you can take control of your body and achieve your dreams for good. So read this book, apply the principles, and lose the fat.

Thanks again for purchasing this book, I hope you enjoy it!

# Chapter 1 - The Truth About Weight Loss

If you have ever thought about losing weight then you have probably researched long and wide in search for the newest craze to shed unwanted fat. If you have been taught by your weight loss experience that skipping solid food and jogging a lot is the only way to get the results that you want, you may be getting the entire weight loss idea wrong.

The truth about weight loss is that it is not what it seems, and people are getting the wrong kind of training when it comes to what they should do to shed extra pounds. Here is the list of some of the things that you thought are the sole reasons why people lose weight.

"Clean" and "detox" food.

Excessive movement and exercise

Staying away from junk food

Lower sugar intake

Lower amount of carbs in the diet

Eating healthy food

Refusing to eat dinner

Doing cardio exercises

Bodybuilding and gaining muscles

Using a much smaller plate

These are just a few examples of an extensive list, but here's the truth about these things. While they may assist in losing weight, they are working on an entirely different concept, and so do you. In fact, you can skip all these and still lose weight, which is something that gym trainers and companies that sell healthy packed juices, pills, and potions do not tell.

Losing weight does not need to be complicated or some sort of rocket science, and even if you do not have the money to enroll in a diet/nutrition program or gym training, the ideal weight is achievable. All you need to do is pay attention to the calories that you take in, it's really that simple! Crazy! Right? After all this time we have been told that all food is not created equal, keep your carbs and fats down and you will lose weight. I won't sit here and tell you that eating vegetables and lean meats is not healthier for you than eating sugar, carbs, and fats, but from a standpoint of losing weight, the most important thing you can do is take in less calories than you burn. That's it. If they exceed the requirement your body needs to function, shed them. In this sense, losing weight is actually very straightforward

## Thanks For Previewing My Exiting Book Entitled:

## "Fat Loss Secrets - No Diets, No Supplements, Just Fat Loss Truth!"

To purchase this book, simply go to the Amazon Kindle store and simply search:

"FAT LOSS SECRETS"

Then just scroll down until you see my book. You will know it is mine because you will see my name "Chris Smith" underneath the title.

Alternatively, you can visit my author page on Amazon to see this book and other work I have done. Thanks so much, and please don't forget your free bonuses

**DON'T LEAVE YET! - CHECK OUT YOUR FREE BONUSES BELOW!**

# Free Bonus Offer: Get Free Access To The www.LiveFitVIP.com VIP Newsletter!

Once you enter your email address you will immediately get free access to this awesome newsletter!

But wait, right now if you join now for free you will also get free access to the "The 7 Keys To Body Transformation" free EBook!

To claim both your FREE VIP NEWSLETTER MEMBERSHIP and your FREE BONUS EBook on THE 7 KEYS TO BODY TRANSFORMATION!

Just Go To:

## www.liveFitVIP.com

www.ingramcontent.com/pod-product-compliance
Lightning Source LLC
Chambersburg PA
CBHW072254310526
45795CB00011B/1103